HOMOEOPATHY
and
IMMUNIZATION

T0316142

compiled by
LESLIE J. SPEIGHT

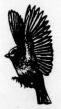

THE C. W. DANIEL COMPANY LTD
1 CHURCH PATH, SAFFRON WALDEN,
ESSEX CB10 1JP, ENGLAND

First Edition 1982
Second Edition 1983
Reprinted 1985
Third Edition 1987
Reprinted 1995

The Random House Group Limited supports The Forest Stewardship
Council (FSC®), the leading international forest certification organisation.
Our books carrying the FSC label are printed on FSC® certified paper.
FSC is the only forest certification scheme endorsed by the leading
environmental organisations, including Greenpeace. Our
paper procurement policy can be found at
www.randomhouse.co.uk/environment

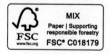

Printed and bound in Great Britain by Clays Ltd, St Ives PLC

ISBN 0 85032 199 9

Set by MS Typesetting, Castle Camps, Cambridge

INTRODUCTION

The increasing public awareness of the dangers associated with some immunizations is arousing great apprehension in many parents. They are questioning the long term effects in spite of the widely recommended procedures by health authorities and doctors.

Many years ago Dr. J. Compton Burnett, a famous homoeopathic doctor, wrote a book entitled 'Vaccinosis' in which he pointed out the ill effects and dangers of vaccination. Since that time immunizations have become commonplace on the assumption that they can prevent the development of a disease. It must be borne in mind, however, that there is no proof that any individual will develop it in the first place.

Statistics are often produced purporting to show that the incidence of a disease has decreased after the introduction of immunization, but diseases have a habit of running in cycles and there is always the possibility of a decrease coinciding with the use of the alleged immunizing agent.

The body has a built-in immunity system and if this is strengthened by good food and satisfactory living conditions, it can play an important role in resisting any epidemic and, in fact, any disease which might attack those who ignore these important factors.

Occasionally there is a report of irreparable damage caused by immunization. Minor effects are not publicised even if they are recognised as being the result of the innoculation which introduces foreign matter into the body.

In homoeopathy there is no immunization as such, but there are remedies that can build up immunity to infections. They can also act as curative agents where a disease has developed. These remedies carry no risk of detrimental effects, they are absolutely safe.

Dr. A. Pulford wrote 'No disease will arise without an existing predisposition to that disease. It is the absence of the predisposition to any particular disease that makes us immune to it. Homoeopathy alone is capable of removing these predispositions.'

The homoeopathic prophylaxis will immunize for 3 to 4 weeks so it should be repeated at the outbreak of another epidemic.

Dr. Dorothy Shepherd states that a homoeopathic preparation of the whooping cough bacillus was administered daily for two weeks to 364 cases after contact with the disease and not one child developed whooping cough. Another homoeopathic physician gave Lathyrus Sativa to 82 people who were in close proximity to the suspect area of poliomyelitis with 12 people being direct contacts. There were 63 children and 19 adults in the group and not one developed the disease.

CHICKEN POX

Early symptoms are an eruption on the trunk, chest and back spreading to the arms and face, usually thicker on the shoulders and upper arms than on wrists and hands. More on thighs than on legs and feet.

Fresh crops of spots appear every two days before or simultaneously with a rise in temperature. There are clear blisters on the skin together with dried up crusts and scabs.

Homoeopathic Prophylaxis

VARICELLA 30, one pill or tablet at 4 hourly intervals for 3 doses in one day. Then one dose weekly while there is a risk of infection.

CHOLERA

This is a disease in which homoeopathy has achieved great success. The death rate under orthodox treatment is very high and statistics giving comparisons of the mortality under the two systems emphasize the superiority of homoeopathic treatment. The early symptoms are usually painless diarrhoea accompanied by sudden prostration and sudden coldness.

Homoeopathic Prophylaxis

RUBINI'S CAMPHOR, 2 or 3 drops on a piece of sugar once or twice a day (it can cause nausea if taken in water).

In addition one or two drops of CUPRUM ACETICUM 3x in a little water may be given night and morning where a person is much exposed to the disease.

Under the heading 'Prevention' Dr. John H. Clarke in his 'Prescriber' says "Wear near the skin a plate of copper (6 in. by 4, for a man of large size; 5 in. by 3 for a small man, and for a woman; 4 in. by 2 for children). Let it be fastened round the waist by straps attached to longitudinal slits cut in the ends of the plate, which should be oval. Let the plate rest in front of the abdominal wall and let it be made slightly concave, so as to adapt itself to the shape of the body. The plate should be worn day and night. It may be cleaned from time to time by rubbing with vinegar."

Where this disease is prevalent hygiene is most important. Rooms should be dry, clean and well aired. Exposure to cold and wet should be avoided.

As homoeopathic treatment is so successful in dealing with this very serious ailment it is always wise to consult a homoeopathic doctor if cholera is suspected.

Dr. Shepherd mentions three 'classic' remedies – Camphor, Cuprum and Veratrum alb., which have proved invaluable when prescribed according to the symptoms. There are, however, other remedies that must be considered when treating this disease.

DIPHTHERIA

Commences with a sore throat and the tonsils and larynx become involved. The membrane of the throat has a glistening gelatinous appearance, the breath has a sickening smell, there is headache and a general feeling of malaise.

Any suspicion of paralysis should be reported to a doctor immediately.

One source of information states that the vaccine seems to be very effective but that, in very rare instances, may cause polio. Another says there is some doubt about its efficacy.

Homoeopathic Prophylaxis

DIPHTHERINUM 30, one pill or tablet at 4 hourly intervals for 3 doses in one day. Then one dose weekly while there is a risk of infection.

Dr. Grimmer, a famous homoeopathic physician, recommended PYROGEN. If the first mentioned remedy is not available immediately take this in the same dosage.

GERMAN MEASLES

Children with this disease display mild symptoms of fever, rash and tiredness. The risk of serious complications is rare.

A significant proportion of mothers who had this complaint during the first three months of pregnancy often produced babies with deformities, eye defects, deafness and mental retardation.

In addition to the protection of children, women of child-bearing age are often given the vaccine if they haven't adequate antibodies in their blood. The vaccine can cause a rash, swollen lymph nodes and pains in the joints, usually between 2 and 10 weeks after the immunization.

Homoeopathic Prophylaxis

RUBELLA 30, one pill or tablet at 4 hourly intervals for 3 doses in one day. Subsequently one dose weekly if there is still risk of infection.

If Rubella is not available immediately take PULSATILLA 12 or 30 in the same dosage.

INFLUENZA

When there is an epidemic of this common trouble take one pill or tablet of INFLUENZINUM 30 night and morning for 3 days. Repeat at weekly intervals while there is a risk.

Some homoeopathic chemists offer two homoeopathic remedies in combination – *Influenzinum* and *Bacillinum* – which seems to be effective. They would advise regarding dosage.

MEASLES

A highly contagious disease characterised by cold symptoms, cough, irritation of the eyes and high fever. A rash appears on the fourth day of the illness. There can be complications such as ear infections, pneumonia and infection of the lymph nodes.

There has been an impressive decline in this complaint since the introduction of the vaccine but there is statistical evidence showing that many cases occur after the vaccination. Some children develop a fever and there are reports of severe reactions of the central nervous system in a few instances.

Martin Weitz in 'Health Shock' states 'Strong reactions of the vaccine are not uncommon. In one survey 32 per cent of children had a general reaction (such as fever and skin rash), which was severe in 6 per cent. But the risk of neurological disorders, i.e. brain damage, is very low according to an American survey of 51 million children vaccinated. It occurred about once in every 600,000 cases. It should not be given to children sensitive to egg protein or those with a history of convulsions, TB or cancer.'

Homoeopathic Prophylaxis

MORBILLINUM 30, one pill or tablet at 4 hourly intervals for 3 doses in one day. Then one dose weekly until the trouble has passed.

If only the 12th potency is available give in the same dosage. In the 200th potency this remedy should be taken once a week for 3 doses.

If the above mentioned is not at hand PULSATILLA 12 or 30 should be given as prescribed for *Morbillinum* 12 and 30.

In many cases *Morbillinum* will help to clear any after effects of measles.

MUMPS

A highly contagious disease commencing with a fever associated with the parotid gland. In addition there is headache and tiredness. Within 24 hours there is earache near the lobe of the ear and the next day the salivary glands in front of the ear become swollen. Pain during mastication and on opening of the mouth. The illness runs its course within 6 days.

In adults there can be orchitis, inflammation of the testicles, ovaries etc. These troubles occur much less frequently in children.

The vaccine seems to give immunity in a very high percentage of cases.

Homoeopathic Prophylaxis

PAROTIDINUM 30 one pill or tablet at 4 hourly intervals for 3 doses in one day.

For the after effects of mumps *Pilocarpine* 6 night and morning should be given for a few days but stopped as soon as an improvement commences and not repeated unless the symptoms recur.

POLIO

The incidence of this much feared disease has decreased dramatically and the vaccine has, apparently, brought about this decline. However, it seems that there are risks; pregnant women should not be vaccinated as it causes a 20% increase in the risk of stillbirths during the first four months of pregnancy.

Polio should always be under the care of a doctor (homoeopathic if possible).

Dr. Grimmer recommends *Lathyrus Sativus* 30 or 200 once every three weeks during an epidemic and he claims that there will be no case of paralysis.

Another homoeopathic remedy that seems to cover the symptoms of polio is *Gelsemium*.

SCARLET FEVER

There are very few cases but the onset of this very contagious disease is abrupt, commencing with vomiting, fever and sore throat. The mucous membrane of the throat is bright red, the tongue is furred with enlarged inflamed papillae showing through the white edges. A skin rash appears within 24 hours with bright red face and it spreads all over the body.

If neglected there can be serious complications but homoeopathy has several most effective remedies and it is advisable to consult a homoeopathic physician as soon as the trouble is suspected.

Homoeopathic Prophylaxis

SCARLATINUM 30, one pill or tablet at 4 hourly intervals for 3 doses in one day. Then one dose at weekly intervals for 3 weeks.

SMALL-POX

The first symptoms are severe backache, intense headache and fever. Also a dirty tongue and deranged stomach. At the commencement the eruption is similar to that of measles but if the finger is passed over the skin there is a feeling – as if fine shot were under the skin.

Homoeopathic Prophylaxis

VARIOLINUM 6 or 30, one pill or tablet night and morning during the trouble. An alternative remedy is MALANDRINUM 30 in the same dosage.

TYPHOID

Caused mainly by lack of cleanliness and bad sanitation. The utmost care should be exercised when handling food – the hands should be scrupulously clean and all food in shops and in the home should be covered to prevent flies contaminating it. Lavatories used by sufferers should be thoroughly disinfected and in places where water is suspect it is advisable to drink only the bottled variety.

Homoeopathic Prophylaxis

TYPHOIDINUM 30, one pill or tablet at 4 hourly intervals for three doses in a day. This may be continued throughout the epidemic.

TYPHUS

Another dirt disease which is usually controlled by cleanliness. Can be passed from one sufferer to another by carrier lice.

Cleanliness is of paramount importance; infected rooms should be disinfected and re-papered.

Homoeopathic Prophylaxis

All the authorities consulted stress the importance of cleanliness and omit to mention remedies. However, one reliable source recommends HYOSCYAMUS or BAPTISIA. One pill or tablet of either in the 12th potency, night and morning, should be taken for several days.

Repeat if considered advisable.

WHOOPING COUGH

An infectious disease of childhood which can sometimes have alarming symptoms. Usually the child appears to have a cold followed by violent coughing for four to six weeks. This mainly occurs in infants and young children.

Deaths are usually due to complicating respiratory troubles. Pneumonia is responsible for a very high proportion of deaths in children under three years of age.

There was a great reduction in the mortality from this disease before the vaccine was introduced. There is conflicting evidence regarding the results of immunization, one report mentions that of 85 fully immunized children at least 46 developed whooping cough.

Homoeopathic Prophylaxis

Immediately there is any risk of contact give one pill or tablet of PERTUSSIN 30 night and morning once a week for 6 to 8 weeks.

PLEASE READ THESE NOTES

When it is impossible to administer a pill or tablet dissolve one pill or crushed tablet in a small wineglass of cold water and give a teaspoonful as a dose.

It is unnecessary to give more than one pill or tablet as a dose although more will do no harm.

Do not repeat the suggested dose unless absolutely necessary as the medicines can work in the body for a considerable time and too frequent repetition can interfere with the curative action.

Homoeopathic medicines are produced by potentisation which renders them sensitive to strong sunlight, odours etc. They should be stored in a cool, dark place away from strong perfumes, scented soap, lipstick, peppermint etc.

When taking the medicines refrain from coffee and strong drinks such as peppermint tea.

Pills and tablets should be allowed to dissolve under the tongue and not be washed down with liquid.

Combinations of homoeopathic medicines are often offered as specifics for a variety of ailments but they cannot be truly homoeopathic as the basic principle of homoeopathy is to individualize. The remedy that has produced similar symptoms in a healthy person must be given. The name of the disease is not important in this scientific method of treatment, except for convenience in describing the patient's condition. When a combination of remedies is given without success homoeopathy is often condemned as useless, a totally unfair assessment.

This small booklet deals only with remedies that act as prophylactics but, at all times, it is advisable to consult a competent homoeopath as soon as trouble is suspected. Homoeopathy can not only act as a preventative but as a most efficient curative method in all ailments, even those deep-seated troubles often considered incurable by other means.

Remember that medicine cannot eradicate symptoms caused by unwise actions such as smoking, poor food, lack of exercise, excessive drinking of alcohol, lack of fresh air etc.

The preparation of homoeopathic medicines is a job for the specialist and, in consequence, it is advisable, at all times, to obtain remedies from a reputable homoeopathic pharmacy.

Most homoeopathic pharmacies supply cases containing ten or twelve bottles of any selected remedies. I have just received one from Ainsworth's Homoeopathic Pharmacy, 38 New Cavendish Street, London, W1M 7LH containing Varicella 30, Diphtherinum 30, Rubella 30, Influenzinum 30, Morbillinum 30, Parotidinum 30, Scarlatinum 30, Pertussin 30, Arnica 30 and Nux Vomica 30.

Arnica should be in every home and given in any accident (it not only deals with bruising but removes the shock, which is so important), overtiredness from excessive exertion, sprains, after tooth extraction and operations.

Nux Vomica gives great relief to people who over-eat and over indulge in alcohol—it clears up 'morning after the night before' feeling very quickly. It has many uses which are given in any materia medica.

When ordering a case of medicines the remedies and potencies should be named.

I hope this small work will be of help to many and save much suffering.

Leslie J. Speight

P.S. There is no standard dosage in homoeopathy. Those who wish to take additional precautions could supplement the suggested dosage by taking one pill or tablet of the same remedy on three consecutive days and repeat this at 3, 6, 9 or 12 monthly intervals.

THE FOLLOWING BOOKS ARE RECOMMENDED FOR THOSE WISHING FOR MORE KNOWLEDGE ABOUT HOMOEOPATHY

HOMOEOPATHY IN EPIDEMIC DISEASES by Dr. Dorothy Shepherd. Enables those far from homoeopathic help to deal with epidemic diseases.

HOMOEOPATHY, A GUIDE TO NATURAL MEDICINE by Phyllis Speight. Excellent for those with no knowledge of the subject.

PUDDEPHATT'S PRIMERS by Noel Puddephatt, revised and re-arranged by Phyllis Speight. Originally three small booklets entitled 'First Steps to Homoeopathy', 'How To Find The Correct Remedy' and 'The Homoeopathic Materia Medica, How It Should be Studied'.

ARNICA THE WONDER HERB by Phyllis Speight. Probably the best ambassador for homoeopathy, giving details of the most commonly used remedy in a great number of everyday troubles.

A STUDY COURSE IN HOMOEOPATHY by Phyllis Speight and THE PRINCIPLES & ART OF CURE BY HOMOEOPATHY by Dr. H. A. Roberts. These two works studied together give a deep understanding of the basis of homoeopathy.

All of the above are available from The C. W. Daniel Company Ltd.